I0500812

Know More, Look Lovelier

Olukunmi Fasina

Contents

1. Acknowledgement
2. Preface
3. Your Body
4. Your mind.
5. Food.
6. Exercises.
7. Destiny.
8. Conclusion.

Acknowledgements

My heartfelt gratitude to:

The members of my family especially Anuoluwa and Ibukun.

Dr. Mike Oye, for sharing his wealth of experience.

Mr. Uju Onyechere, for helping to make my dreams a reality.

Mrs Olajide, for painstakingly proofreading this book.

I appreciate you all.

Preface

In life, everybody wants to look lovely whether they accept that fact or not. Some had the habit of habit of looking lovely inculcated into them early in life while some had to learn even after becoming full grown. Whichever way we all love to look lovely and be appreciated by others. How often we love to hear, 'you are look lovely' kids inclusive. But to look lovely is not a kid's job. Ask some people who have tried to loss real excess weight before and you would be amazed at what some of them go through.

A lot of people work very hard, but neglect their health. They forget that the strength you expend on a daily basis come from what you put inside. I mean what is the essence of having a lot of money but you can't enjoy it because the body is no longer healthy and a very large chunk of the money is actually spent to keep you alive.

I am quite sure you really desire that your stay on this side should be a memorable one not just for you, but also as a reference point for generations after you. To do that, some vital things would have to be put in place. There is a secret on how to 'know more and look lovelier.' What is it that as you know more of it and it makes you look lovelier? It's nothing more than **applied information** or knowledge (the useful one of course). Did you notice the word 'applied?' That's because of lot of people have so many useful information at their fingertips but fail to apply them to make their life better. So also will you have wasted your time and money if you fail to apply whatever information you get from this book. I encourage you to take every step necessary as you read. Don't just acquire the information, please apply it. So without wasting time, let's

set the ball rolling. Welcome
on board.

YOUR BODY

The body of man is what houses the wonderful systems the Creator has given man. It plays a very important role because without it, you won't belong to this planet. The body should be handled with care if you want it to be around for long and function properly. It is said that being healthy is not just the absence of disease. So don't think you hundred percent okay simply because you are not combating any disease. Let's now discuss about your body.

Have you ever appreciated that body? Do you marvel at how every part has been created and the function of each? If you do not appreciate your body in its entirety, how can you take good care of it? When you do not know the purpose of a thing, its abuse is inevitable. If you cherish your body, would you want to fill it with things that will harm it, make it weak or deteriorate it? Will you allow just anybody to handle it anyhow? I'm sure your answer is a big NO. Therefore, your body should always be handled with care and treated courteously, by you first and then others.

How do you take care of your body? You need to take your bath regularly, preferably morning and night, and apply cream. Brush your teeth, first thing in the morning and last thing at night. Put on clean under-wears and well ironed cloths. Make sure you cut your finger and toe nails regularly. Another thing to take good care of is your bathroom and toilet. Ensure they are always clean and make use of disinfectants and air fresheners to make the place really lovely. Also where you sleep is very, very important. Make sure it is neat, tidy and well ventilated. It should also be free from dangerous insects, most especially mosquitoes. The kitchen and the other rooms in the house and the environment you keep your body in generally must be always clean because all these are essential to the well being of your body.

When you take good care of your body, it will serve you better and last longer. Handle it carelessly and you cut it short. We were taught in science that the human body is divided into the brain, the thorax and the abdomen. The three main systems connecting all these are the nervous system, the blood system and the lymphatic system. I am not going to bother you with scientific terms so just relax. When all these systems are in good condition, you can be very sure that your body will be very healthy and good. The purpose of this book is to further enlighten you on how to take good care of your body because you have a definite purpose to fulfil on earth. No other person will start the assignment unless you ignite it. The elements of nature will not respond to other peoples' call to do the assignment because they have been commanded and ordained to respond to you ALONE. Did you read that? So, you can't afford to belittle or mesmerise your body. It's yours. God gave you. So, keep it.

Well, are you reading this and the thought "you don't know the type of body I have" is passing through your mind? Not to worry, simply be grateful that you are alive and once you are alive, there is hope and you will certainly fulfil your destiny. Have you heard of Helen Keller, Dr. Glenn Cunningham or Ludwig Van Beethoven, just to mention a few? It was said that Beethoven wrote some of his greatest masterpieces when he lost his hearing. If they were successful despite their challenges, then certainly yours won't be an exception.

I'd tell you how adversity had helped someone I know. While in school, he never knew he could write until he had a lot of problems with his academics and he felt he was no good. It was then that he started writing just to console himself and it was there that someone encouraged him to start writing to help people based on what he had also experienced. Also, something else came along, he developed a deep flair for those who had written themselves off or people had written off because of what had happened to them. Today, helping such people he said has made him a fulfilled person.

If you are however still not contented, then talk to the one who gave you the body. Have faith like Helen Keller and Dr. Glenn Cunningham and you will also be a wonder to the world. We should be grateful for adversity anyway because Horace (65-8BC) said "adversity has the effect of eliciting talents, which in prosperous circumstances would have lain dormant".

To wrap it up friend, learn to be grateful that you have a body no matter what anyone thinks, it's your body not theirs, so you have a duty towards it. Where you fit in, they can't fit in and where you stand, others may not have what it takes. So, appreciate your body because without it you'd no longer be here and always remember that you cannot become whatsoever you desire to be without a body. In other words, accept and love your body. It is simply unique.

YOUR MIND

The human mind is the seat of emotions. That is where you reason out things. That is also where you are either made or marred. Your mind can be an instrument of developing good things or destruction. It all depends on you. Great or small minds are not born rather they are made. How do know I know myself you may wish to ask? Your thoughts - your thoughts make you. What do feed your mind on? Your mind is your life wire because your thinking affects how you behave (your attitude) and your behaviour gradually becomes your character. If you feed your mind with dirty, ungodly or evil things, then you can't enjoy life. Even if you live long, it's going to be a bad life which will leave a bitter memory behind.

Is your mind filled with fear? You know what, fear has torment. It is a powerful, paralyzing emotion. You must get rid of it by facing it; doing that which you afraid to do. When your mind is not properly oriented and healthy, you will go through life as a casualty. I know an individual who because he failed some core exams, became bitter with God, gave in to self pity which made inferiority complex set in. He said it took me some years to get over the whole issue because he already had concluded in his mind that he was no good. He would have gone through life as a casualty, had he not discovered that my mind needed healing and that nobody was going to do it for him, except himself. So, he took up the challenge (he actually testified that it wasn't really easy) but since he was determined, he made progress and he's still making progress by the grace of God.

You can never be the best you were created to be if

your mind is sick. Have you seen people who have everything it takes to live comfortably and yet pretend to be happy or are battling with one disease or the other and are not simply themselves? Whereas on the other hand, you have people who don't have much but are happy, friendly and may not encounter any terminal disease? What do you think is the secret of the latter group? They have simply discovered the positive power of the mind and so they are enjoying it. To enjoy life, your mind must be at peace and undergo stead growth. You must make a conscious effort to guard your mind from things that will prevent its expansion from becoming deep and fruitful. Your mind is the seat of emotion, so allow faith, determination, good ideas, self-discipline, trust, good dreams, love, honesty, humility(to mention a few) to thrive in it. Say no to worry, depression, pride, ignorance, unforgiveness and greed. Never give them a chance. They have just a singular mission, to steal your joy and kill it if you don't resist them. Joy is related to strength. When you have joy, you have strength oozing out of you. Worry, depression, pride, ignorance, unforgiveness and greed sap your strength.

Dear friend, you need strength to achieve your dreams. Learn to encourage yourself even when nobody does. The story was told about a man who encouraged himself when all hope was gone. He had lost everything he could call his - wives and children included. Even his friends were bitter against him. But because he encouraged himself the right way, he recovered every single thing he had lost. If you wouldn't consider it a waste of time, please read the whole account in 1Kings, Chapter 30. Don't sit down and weep. Weeping, worrying changes nothing. Although our nature makes us cry a times, it shouldn't turn to self pity. You are responsible for who are. Nobody will make you, you will make yourself. Your mind is you. So, to enjoy life and live long, your mind must be sharp and active. Think good thoughts. How do you do that? Read good books; inspirational, educative, motivational e.t.c. Keep the right company - people that have a focus, creative, optimistic, lovers of success. Watch the right programs on the T.V; computer/internet and the satellite. I said the right programs because these three have done more harm than good. If you train your mind in the good path - the path of life, then you will know how to refuse evil or contaminating sight when you see one.

Who is your hero? Who do you pattern your life after? This actually matters a lot. Who you see is who you become. Before you choose your hero, why don't you find out how he lived, his achievements and exit? If he's still living, is he worthy to be your hero? There's a way that your thoughts affect your body. When your mind is clouded, you can't think straight, you get stressed up and before you know it, headache sets in. When this gradually becomes a way of life, and it's not quickly checked and attended to, frustration sets in, you become someone else and once there is no ease in the body chemical metabolism, various diseases set in. You start spending money on drugs, your health deteriorates and before you know it you've got what you didn't bargain for. Also, you've got to be current. Someone said, "being current is the currency of time". To do that, take time to attend seminars that you feel will make you better in any area of your life that you think needs improvement. As a matter of fact, we all need to improve upon every aspect of our life because the day a man stops learning, he starts dying. So if you don't want to die yet, learn something new that is good, inspiring and soul lifting.

When you think good things, you see, hear, do, have, and love good things. Your thinking determines where you would get to in life. It is said that the battle is first won in the mind. If you can win the battle in your mind, then nothing can subdue you. So make up your mind to think good thoughts. When situations arise that you can do nothing about, simply keep your cool and think of something good that can come out of it. Even the Bible encourages us not to worry about tomorrow. You have today, so use it and only prepare for tomorrow, not worry about it because you don't have power over it.

Take life easy. And lest I forget, there is one more thing I should say. Can you guess? It starts with L. It is laughter, real laughing. I laugh a lot. Learn to laugh heartily. Have a sense of humour. Laugh with your spouse, children, family, friends, business associates etc. Laugh at your mistakes too. To this end, René's Descartes said "Cogito ergo sum" *that is*, I think, therefore I am. The very existence of man is predicted on his ability to process thought. The potential of the human mind is beyond enormous. It is unfathomable. Research has shown that only 10% of the mind is used in any lifetime. The mind is a terrible thing to waste. I am not going to waste mine so what about you? Remember, as a man thinks in his heart, so he is. Abundant life is available to you. Do not do anything to deprive yourself of this gift God has given you. You were created to dominate, so do not be dominated. Find your place and keep it.

FOOD

Food is popularly called the friend of the skin. I am quite sure you would have expected me to start with food. Well, if you must know, your body and the mind would not appreciate the food if they have been abused. I have seen some people's body reject food simply because their minds were wounded. Alright, so let's talk about food. You are what you eat. You either eat or die. That is the truth and what you feed your body with determines how effective and lasting it would be. If you feed it with junk, that is the type of body you'd have and if you feed it with good and healthy food, then you have a good and healthy body. A lot of us eat what we can find but it shouldn't be. Don't just eat for eating sake rather, eat to stay alive. Don't eat for pleasure, but for strength. It's when you are alive that you can make those ideas a reality.

Before we talk about foods to eat, let's talk about how to eat. When you eat, don't do any other thing. Eating time talk is not a time for discussion, cracking jokes or watching the TV. Concentrate on your food and enjoy it first. Always eat in a very relaxed atmosphere. Don't eat in a rush because it leads to indigestion which makes the blood stay in your brain and not your stomach.

Never overeat. Once you eat and you are about to be filled, that's when to stop. Digestion starts from the mouth and the more you chewed the better the digestion. The chemicals that digest food in the body are called enzymes and they work best in concentrated environment. Therefore, when you eat, don't drink. Preferably, drink water one hour before or after eating. Due to our drinking habit, man has had to battle with so many diseases. We need to watch it. The heat of your stomach, salivary gland and intestine are very important. So, never overeat.

Overeating brings a problem to the digestive system. Don't eat deep into the night and go to bed about thirty minutes after. Indigestion may occur and this is one of the reasons people fall sick and may even lead to death. Before we move on, let me chip in this. Of the three meals in the day, the breakfast is the most important. You need to break the fast once hunger bites; and no hot or cold food please. I didn't know these facts too until recently, and I've been practising these principles too. Though a time, I fall short of them, most especially, not drinking during meals but I've adapted now. One thing that has helped is having my bottle of water with me always when I go to places (don't drink water just anywhere, it's dangerous to your health) and I have to drink before I get back home.

That done, let's check what happens after the food has been digested. The intestines comprise both the small and large intestines. You have mainly food waste in the large intestine. It does not digest the waste but prepare it for evacuation. The large intestine is where most diseases arise from. Diseases are caused mainly by poisonous chemicals in the body. Anyone who can manage the large intestine effectively is able to overcome about 90% of body diseases. In the large intestine, two things take place. Firstly, extra water is absorbed back into the blood again by the walls of the large intestine and secondly, the solid or semi solid substance left is pushed down by rhythmic reaction towards the rectum in readiness to be expelled from the body. This elimination is part of detoxification, which is known as defecation. This is the most important aspect of detoxification for keeping the body healthy. In the large intestine, there are thousands of different useful bacteria. Most of them help in making sure most of the wastes there are processed for defecation. When a person refuses to go to toilet, fermentation (decay) begins to take place. Secondly, the walls of the intestine continue to absorb water from the faeces, and then the faeces become caked. Parts of these faeces now stick to the walls of the large intestine and this leads to the production of dangerous gases e.g. hydrogen sulphide, nitrogen(ii) oxide and nitrogen(i) oxide that are absorbed into the blood stream. When these gases are absorbed into the blood stream, they form dangerous acids that are toxic to the body. The whole body starts feeling pains and these cause diseases like cancer, tumours, boils, high blood pressure, arthritis, oedema, e.t.c. Constipation also sets in. The caked faeces cause lacerations on the rectum, colon and anus. This leads to diseases like piles and haemorrhoids. External infection can also set in. Lack of drinking enough water can also cause constipation. It is proposed that every human being should drink about eight glasses of water a day.

It is however advisable to eliminate twice a day, first in the morning and last thing at night. When you put all these things into practice, your health will definitely improve and you will be all over the place full of energy. Shall we now talk about the right type of food the body needs to be healthy?

We need vitamins, amino acids and minerals in order to be very healthy. They are very essential in the diet we take. A diet is a combination of all types of food. A balanced diet does not mean it should be in one plate or meal. Rather, it should be a diet for a day. From nutrition diet research, you can have a diet in a week. It makes the alimentary canal very effective. You have thorough digestion, absorption and assimilation. You can make your cycle 2 or 4 days or a week. For example, on Monday, eat carbohydrates, Tuesday, vegetables, Wednesday, protein

Thursday, fruits, etc. Some foods that are very good that you can base your diet on include oatmeal, sweet potatoes, wild rice, brown rice, yam, lima beans, black beans, tomatoes, all dark vegetables, mango, avocado pear, grapes, apples, oranges, grapefruit, milk (whole or skimmed), yogurt that has not been sweetened. These foods do not trigger insulin, while some of the dangerous ones are white bread, Irish baked potato, ordinary rice, polished rice, black tea (any tea without milk) French fries, rice cakes, crackers, spaghetti etc. Other good sources include whole grains, egg yolk, fish, onions, lettuce, cabbage, corn, brewers yeast or normal yeast, oyster, shrimps, lobster, crabs, sesame seeds, cashew, fish liver oil, pawpaw, cucumber, spinach, soya beans, mushrooms, organ meats, poultry, walnuts, bell pepper, garlic, ginger, banana, honey etc.

Tips To Remember

- Drastically reduce the amount of palm oil and coconut oil you take. The best oils are olive oil, sunflower oil, and beniseed oil. Use small quantities however.

- Food preservatives are dangerous, so avoid them. All polished food, refined sugar, bottled soft drinks, alcohol should be avoided. (You can use brown sugar instead). Apart from the fact that they don't supply the body with vitamins and minerals, they deplete the body of the ones already there, which can lead to hormonal imbalance.

- Avoid urine therapy.
- As much as possible, avoid fat, margarine, and animal fat.
- Eat food that contains fibre.
- Take enough water. Water is necessary for high metabolism.

- Avoid fried foods because they deplete the body of vitamin E.

EXERCISES

The well being of the body is not complete without exercise. This is because during exercise the heart beats faster, and in this way every part of the body gets a better supply of blood. During exercise one breathes oftener, and in this way every part of the body gets a more abundant supply of oxygen. The mind becomes dull if the muscles of the body are not exercised. If one desires to have a good memory and be able to study diligently and learn rapidly, one must exercise the muscles of the body daily.

The work of the muscles is to move limbs or other parts of the body. It is not only when we move about that the muscles have work to do, even when standing still it requires the constant contraction of many muscles to keep the body erect. Many people while standing or sitting, allow the muscles of the back to relax, the result is that the back becomes humped and the shoulders droop forward. This is not only unsightly, but also causes the walls of the chest to press in on the lungs so that deep breathing is interfered with. When sitting on a chair or at a study desk, the body should be erect. When standing, stand as tall as possible. The front wall of the abdomen should not be allowed to protrude, but should be drawn in toward the back.

The importance of sitting and standing erect cannot be too strongly emphasized. We may make our blood ever so pure by supplying it with proper food, but if habitual incorrect posture cramps the blood vessels so that life giving fluid cannot circulate in all parts of the body, ill health is sure to result.

When God created man's body, He knew just what the body required to keep it strong and healthy; and so He not only provided food to nourish the body, but He also made provision that man must work and exercise his body in order to secure food.

The one most needed is aerobic type of exercise. Ten minutes of this everyday improves health. Examples include running, brisk walking, jumping the rope, climbing stairs quickly, jogging, and swimming. Another type is stretching exercises like sit up, press up, e.t.c. which strengthens the muscles.

The mechanism of breathing is extremely also very important for health. Deep rhythmic breathing is very healthy and so make sure you practice it always because it helps to eliminate dangerous gases. It has also been proved that gardening and walking helps. So, start practising if you haven't been doing it.

Tip

Vacation should be consciously integrated into the year's program so that awareness is already there to go on break.

DESTINY

No matter whom you are, where you are, what you are going through, there is a definite assignment awaiting you. We all have a definite task to fulfil on earth. You have yours, I have mine. It is the duty of each individual to seek it out. God has endowed each of us with talents, ideas and dreams which would help us to follow the steps towards fulfilling our destiny. Pause for a moment and imagine how the world would be without Alexander Graham Bell, who invented the telephone, Ed Roberts, who created the world's first commercially successful personal computer, Mr. Honda, whose corporation is considered as one of the biggest car making empires in Japan, outselling all but Toyota in the United States. What of people like Shakespeare, Plato, Socrates, Aristotle and others? They all contributed their quota in their respective generations. But mind you, we wouldn't be reading about them today if they hadn't taken good care of their health. I should say they were more fortunate because most of the junk people feed themselves with now weren't available then. On a second thought however, I would rather say they were men who disciplined themselves to accomplish their purpose on earth. They just didn't live;

they had a clearly defined reason for living.

It has been said that the grave is the richest place, all because you have a lot of untapped potentials buried there. Don't send yourself to an early grave because of your eating habit. When you know that you are here for a definite purpose, it will certainly affect all you do. Think about it.

It is only when you are alive doing what you love best that you really actually exist.

Your family, the society and the world at large needs you. If it's only a life you can affect positively while you are here, it is enough. That one soul might be the one destined to reach millions of souls. You can't afford to fail. Remember, it's only when you are alive and healthy that you can actually maximise your God given potentials. You will succeed. Stay blessed.

CONCLUSION

On a final note, I would like to share with you the words of these wise men. 'In his biography D.L. Moody, The American Evangelist, by Bonnie Harvey, D.L. Moody said "Trust in yourself and you are doomed to disappointment.... , trust in money and you may have it taken from you..., but trust in God and you are never to be confounded in time or eternity". William Webb added "Don't try to hold God's hand; let Him hold yours". Let Him do the holding and you do the trusting.

And from me, always remember that life in the real sense is in donation and not in duration as it is popularly said, so it's not how long you live that actually matters but the various lives you have been able to touch while living. What will you be remembered for? No matter the age one dies, once you have fulfilled your destiny (and you will feel fulfilled if you have), then that's all. There's no point staying around for long doing practically nothing.

There's nothing impossible with God once you set your mind to achieve it. So, if there are habits to correct, please don't hesitate to do so. Go ahead and fulfil your destiny. Stay blessed.

www.ingramcontent.com/pod-product-compliance
Lightning Source LLC
Chambersburg PA
CBHW070402290526
45790CB00004B/1599